Dan F

53/54
Exercises
2 Desc 3-7

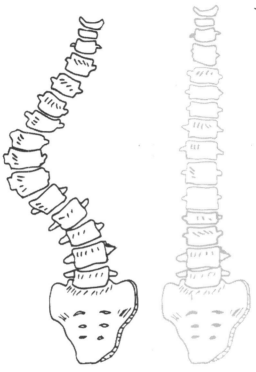

BACK TO
NORMAL

Natural Healing Without
Medications, Injections and Surgery

Back to Normal
© 2016 Chad Madden

Contributors: Dan Hinnerschitz and Joe Hribick
Book & Cover Design: IF Design Graphic Design & Photography, Ida Fia Sveningsson Konsult
Cartoon Images: Randy Glasbergen

ISBN-13: 978-1518712081
ISBN-10: 1518712088

Why Read "Back to Normal"?

This book was written for YOU.

The purpose of this book is to help YOU live a happier and healthier life.

Contained are tools and information to give you a better understanding of the human body and a better understanding of your own body.

As many say, "*Knowledge is power.*"

The more knowledge we have about something, the better we can control that area of our life.

The more knowledge you have about how your body works, the easier it will be to live a healthier life.

If you're suffering with back pain and sciatica...and feel like everyone else gets to live life and have fun while you're sitting on the sideline...

Then read "Back to Normal."

Use it. Gain knowledge. And take control of your body.
Happy healing!

Chad Madden
Physical Therapist

PS - This book was written specifically for back pain and sciatica sufferers looking to heal naturally without medications, injections and surgery.

If at any time while you are going through this book and don't under-stand something...or have a question...you can email me at **chad.madden@maddenpt.com**

Table of Contents

CHAPTER 1   01
The 3 Common Causes of Back Pain and Sciatica

CHAPTER 2   11
What is Pain? Is Pain a Bad Thing...Something That Should
Be Avoided at All Costs? Or is There a Benefit to Feeling Pain?

CHAPTER 3   15
Is There Hope for Back Pain and Sciatica Sufferers?
How We Can Tell if It's Possible that a Person Can Heal
Naturally.

CHAPTER 4   21
What Can You Do?
(Especially When You've "Tried Everything"?!)

CHAPTER 5   27
What is the most common mistake people make in
handling PAIN?

Success Stories   41

Home Exercises   53

A Special Offer   60

About the Authors   61

CHAPTER 1

The 3 Common Causes of Back Pain and Sciatica

Why is it so important to find the exact CAUSE of your back pain?

We see many back pain and sciatica sufferers who've had failed treatment in the past...

Failed surgery...
Failed injections...
No relief with chiropractic care...
And even more pain after Physical Therapy elsewhere...

And most of the time...the sufferer was getting treatment that did not treat the CAUSE of his or her back pain and sciatica.

Does this sound like your back pain and sciatica story too?

So let's take a look at the 3 Most Common Causes of Back Pain and Sciatica...

Read through them and see if one matches up with what you are going through...

And by the way...we see a lot of people who make the error of being fixated on the results of an MRI or X-ray...and will say things like:

1

"But I've already had an MRI or X-ray...I know what's causing my back pain and sciatica..."

I'd encourage those people to keep an open mind...as X-rays and MRIs don't always show the whole picture...

Cause #1 – Arthritis, Stenosis and Disc Degeneration

These 3 are listed together because the way they cause pain is similar...

Have you ever noticed the person leaning on the shopping cart as they walk through the grocery store?

Then there's a good chance you've seen a person with arthritis, stenosis or disc degeneration (often written on X-ray or MRI reports as "DDD").

People suffering with arthritis, stenosis and DDD usually have pain with standing and walking...

They will usually have more than 50 birthday candles on their next birthday cake (50 years of age or older)...

And they get relief when they sit down. They will frequently say, "Let me just sit down for a minute." (Not because they're tired...but because of back and leg pain and discomfort).

In fact, if you've identified with the 3 items above...pain with standing and walking that goes away when you sit down AND you're 50 years of age or older...then there's a 99% chance you have arthritis, stenosis and DDD.

Here's How it Works...

Compared to when you were 18 years old...are you taller now?

Most likely not...

Most of us shrink as we age.

One of the key factors to us shrinking as we age is a decrease in the space between the bones in your back (the bones are called "vertebrae").

So when that happens...the hole where the nerve comes out in the back also shrinks...

So when we bend back...as when we are standing or walking...the hole gets smaller...and puts more pressure on the nerve. When we lean forward...as when we sit down...the hole gets bigger...and takes pressure off of the nerve.

"Is it possible to be normal again if I have arthritis, stenosis or DDD?"

The short answer is YES...

We'll talk more about this later...but first, here's a quick story of someone who was suffering with arthritis and stenosis...

> *I love the one-on-one experience. You are told if you are doing your exercises wrong. I had severe back pain even walking 5 minutes. Now I can walk without any pain. I admit, I was doubtful because I had tried other PT elsewhere & it was not working. I am thrilled that I can avoid more surgery at this point. I will faithfully do the exercises at home. The cards are a great help. All in all, it has been a wonderful experience."*

— **Rachel Springers**

Back Pain and Sciatica Cause #2 - Herniated Discs

Back Pain and Sciatica sufferers from a herniated or slipped disc usually have sharp pain down the back of their leg...

It usually starts in their lower back or butt and can travel down to the back of the knee...the calf...or even into the foot and toes.

(In addition to "sharp pain"...they may also experience numbness, tingling or heaviness in the leg.)

Herniated disc sufferers usually have pain bending forward, twisting, lifting, coughing or sneezing...

Most are 35 years of age and younger...

Usually their pain goes away with standing or bending backwards.

Are herniated discs common?

If you took an MRI of 100 random people WITHOUT back pain...how many would have a disc bulge or herniation on their MRI?

80...80% of people have disc herniations or bulges on an MRI but do NOT have pain...

So this begs the question: "Can you heal a herniated disc?"

We'll talk about that more in a later chapter...but first...

Here's How It Works...

There is a space between the bones in your back.

In this space there is a disc.

The disc acts as a shock absorber to help with the forces in your spine.

The disc is surrounded by a gel-like substance.

This is held together by a wall of fibers.

Due to repeated stress and force (from bending forward and lifting repeatedly...or from a trauma – like a car accident), these fibers can break down.

This allows some of the disc material and gel to push out and put pressure on the nerves in the lower back.

When this happens, the disc can put an increasing amount of pressure on the nerves in the spine which can lead to pain, numbness, tingling and even "heaviness" or weakness in the leg.

When this happens, the back pain and sciatica sufferer can usually take their finger and trace the sciatica nerve down the back of their leg.

This is true "Sciatica."

❝ *When I first started having issues with my lower back and shooting pains down my leg, I was very skeptical about coming to PT. I was at another PT office 2 years ago when the first incident occurred and it was a waste of my time. They didn't listen to what I was trying to tell them about my pain. When I came here to Madden, Dan, Amanda, and Tiffany paid attention when I would tell them about my pain. They made a workout that took my pain away within two weeks. I couldn't be happier with my experience and will be sure to refer anyone I know who needs PT to come to Madden."*

— **Bob D.**

Back Pain and Sciatica Cause #3 – The SI Joint and Pelvis

This is probably the most missed cause of back pain and sciatica that we have seen in our PT clinic...

Why?

Because it's frequently missed on an MRI or X-ray...
Back pain and sciatica sufferers with a problem in their SI joint or pelvis usually have trouble rolling over in bed, getting in and out of a car, walking up and down stairs, sitting for long periods, driving, crossing one leg over the other or getting dressed.

Many will frequently report sharp pain shooting into their groin.

Some may even have problems controlling their bladder...and may experience "leakage".

Sexual activity can be painful.

SI Joint and Pelvic problem sufferers can have pain, numbness, tingling and heaviness into the leg as well...

They might say things like, "One leg feels heavier than the other."

Most report the pain is more of a "broad ache" down the <u>outside of their thigh and leg that wraps around.</u>

And ages?

Well, this is where it gets a bit tricky...

With SI Joint and Pelvic Issues, we've seen 15 year old dancers to 23 year old NFL football players to 37 year old mothers of three to 84 year old retired construction workers who've had this...

Just realize it's common...

And if you've suffered with back pain and sciatica...and have tried treatments which did not work for you...then there's a good chance you could have an underlying SI joint and pelvic problem.

Here's How It Works...

If you look at a stack of block on a table, what's the most important block?

The top block?

If you move the top block, does it affect the other blocks below?

What about the block on bottom?

If you move the block on the bottom...the entire stack comes tumbling down...

Because you took away the foundation of the stack of blocks...

Your back works the same way.

The foundation for the bones in your spine is your pelvis.

There are 3 bones and 3 joints in the pelvis.

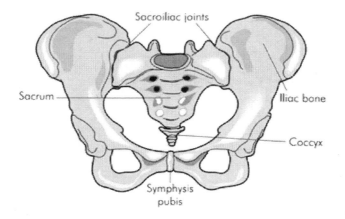

The joint in front is called the "Pubic Symphysis".

The two joints on either side of the tailbone are called "Sacroiliac Joints" or "SI Joints" (for short).

The 3 joints need to be moving and need to be stable for you to move without any pain...and get back to normal.

❝ *Before coming to PT at Madden, there were days I barely could get through the day without wanting to cry from pain. As an OT in pediatrics, my job is for me to be mobile and it was getting increasingly difficult. There were also days where heavy lifting/work caused me difficulty even getting out of bed. Since coming to PT and working with Joe and Michelle, there are days, more so than not, where I think, "I can't believe another day of no pain." They have given me the ability to do my job better, be an active participant in my life, and know what a pain-free life means. The tools they have provided me have made me successful and excited as I continue my life and my passion of working with kids with no pain. I am forever grateful for the wonderful experience. Thank you!"*

— Jamie S.

A Special Offer for You... the Reader of "Back to Normal"

So after reading this first chapter on the 3 Common Causes of Back Pain and Sciatica...do you have a good idea of what the cause of your pain is?

Sometimes this is super easy...

Other times it can be more complicated.

If you're looking for more tools to heal naturally without medications, injections or surgery...send me an email at **chad.madden@maddenpt.com**.

In the subject line write what you think the cause of your pain is. ("Stenosis"; or "Herniated Disc"; or "SI Joint")

Then in the email...let me know why you think that's your cause.

This email account is monitored daily...we will get back to you with some helpful advice as soon as possible.

Cordially,

Chad Madden
Physical Therapist, Back Pain & Sciatica Specialist

CHAPTER 2

What is Pain? Is Pain a Bad Thing... Something That Should Be Avoided at All Costs? Or is There a Benefit to Feeling Pain?

Webster's Dictionary defines pain as a "localized physical suffering associated with bodily disorder (as a disease or an injury)."

Pain originally meant revenge, penalty or punishment.

We feel pain in many ways.

It is a part of our lives.

And while it may not be pleasant and is something to be avoided, how we respond to pain often determines how we feel later on.

As physical therapists, we are experts in helping people handle pain.

When someone comes in suffering from pain, one of the first questions we ask is: "Is pain good or bad?"

Most people answer "Bad".

A small percentage will say pain is a good thing.

They say, "It is a sign, an indicator."

Let's take a look at this...

Our body has five senses:
1. Sight
2. Sound
3. Taste
4. Smell
5. Touch

We see with our eyes. We can see things that are bad and affect us in negative ways. We can receive pleasant sights such as seeing a loved one or a picture of a past family vacation which brings back fond memories.

We hear with our ears. We can hear bad things which disturb us emotionally. We can hear soothing sounds which relax us such as our favorite music.

We taste with the taste buds on our tongue. We can taste things which are bitter such as a lemon. We can taste things which are sweet such as a piece of chocolate.

We smell with our nose. We can smell a bad odor such as a skunk. We can smell something pleasant such as flowers.

We touch with our skin. We can sense heat, cold, pressure, and pain with our skin. Some touch is pleasant such as a massage or a pat on the back. Some sensations are not pleasant such as lower back pain.

So with each sense, there is information being sent to our brain. It may be good or bad or somewhere in between. The information helps us respond and take appropriate action.

What happens when we lose a sense?
Loss of the ability to see is blindness.
Loss of the ability to hear is deafness.

There is a name for a condition in which a person loses their sense of touch. Do you know what it is? Leprosy. A person with leprosy, or leper, suffers nerve damage. This nerve damage prevents them from feeling pain and damage to the body. A healthy person steps on a nail, feels terrible pain, and gets the nail out of their foot. They receive the signal of pain and can take the right action. A person with leprosy, steps on a nail and does not feel pain.

They may continue to walk and cause more damage. They do not feel pain and do not take the right action.

So let us be thankful we can feel pain!

Here's a "Back to Normal" Truth:

Pain is a message with valuable information.

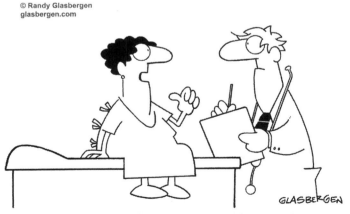

© Randy Glasbergen
glasbergen.com

"You have to learn about thousands of diseases, but
I only have to focus on fixing what's wrong with ME!
Now which one of us do you think is the expert?"

CHAPTER 3

Is There Hope for Back Pain and Sciatica Sufferers? How We Can Tell if It's Possible that a Person Can Heal Naturally.

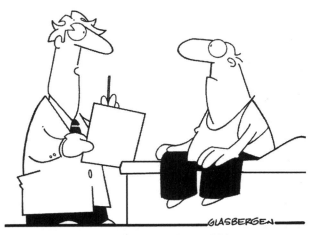

"The good news is, you're the healthiest person I've seen all day. The bad news is, you're the healthiest person I've seen all day."

As a physical therapist, one of the first things we look at in helping someone with back pain and sciatica is the activity which reproduces the pain.

Following is a list of common activities which can make pain worse:

Back Pain and Sciatica

- Sitting
- Standing
- Walking
- Going up or down stairs
- Sleeping
- Getting up in the morning
- Getting dressed

- Leaning forward at a sink
- Golfing
- Lifting
- Running
- Crossing one leg over the other
- Putting shoes or socks on
- Stooping or kneeling

So for you...have you had back pain or sciatica in the past 30 days?

Between 0 and 10 (0 is no pain, 10 is severe pain), what's the WORST your pain has been?

What were you doing when you had that pain?

Is it on the list above?

If so...then we have BAD NEWS...

There's HOPE for you :-)

This brings us to "Back to Normal" Truth #2:

If the pain is <u>reproducible</u>, it is usually <u>reducible</u>.

By "reproducible", we mean when you do an activity, the pain increases. By "reducible", we mean the pain has the potential to decrease…

The good news is that when the pain is reproducible, there is a *CAUSE*. When there is a cause we can handle in PT, there is hope!

Example.

Many people we work with in physical therapy believe that their condition is very rare and hopeless with no chance of healing.

They have been discouraged with failed treatments in the past.

Or they may have seen specialist after specialist, doctor after doctor, or therapist after therapist with no real change in the pain they are feeling.

The same people who feel there is no hope (and think, "I'm the only person suffering with this") are often surprised to learn that their condition is not rare and that we have helped hundreds of people with the same condition in the past year!

A new trend in healthcare is the growing number of people who are seeking treatments without medications, injections and surgery.

They reason the body has a natural ability to heal. They seek ways to increase that ability.

As Physical Therapists, it is our job to help people heal the problem that is causing their back pain and sciatica.

Not all problems causing back pain and sciatica are able to be healed with physical therapy…but there is good news, most problems can be healed with physical therapy treatment.

An example of a problem which cannot heal with PT is cancer. Physical therapists are trained to look for signs of cancer when we are working with a person. One common sign of pain caused by cancer is that regardless of the person's activity, the pain stays about the same.

When a therapist is working with a person whose pain is not reproducible, this is a "red flag." That person needs to be referred back to the family doctor for further testing.

An example of a problem which can heal with PT is a herniated disc. A person with a herniated disc often experiences lower back pain and sciatica (pain shooting down the back of the leg). Pain from a herniated disc is likely to be reproduced with activities involving bending over or bending forward, sitting for long periods of time, lifting, sneezing or coughing.

Again, if the pain is reproducible, it is often reducible...and there is hope.

CHAPTER 4

What Can You Do?
(Especially When You've
"Tried Everything"?!)

Truth #1 is "Pain is a message with valuable information."

Any time in life, when we receive information, we have a choice of what we can do:

1. We can ignore it.
2. We can try to change it or alter it.
3. We can handle it.

Ignoring the pain is the easiest and most common mistake people make. We will explore this more in depth in Chapter 5. For now, understand that ignoring the pain means making no attempt to handle it...usually by making EXCUSES...

Another common mistake people make in handling pain is attempting to change the pain *without addressing the cause*. The person with back pain may take medications to calm down the inflammation...but not the _cause_ of the inflammation. They may take a pain killer to try to block the signal of pain. They may use a heating pad, electrical stimulation, TENS (a small electrical, pain blocking device), or ultrasound to change the pain they are feeling.

Usually, the person trying to alter the sensation of pain may succeed in blocking the pain...for a short time. As long as they fail to address the cause of the pain, once the effects of the heating pad or other temporary help wears off, the pain returns.

If we are looking for long term, permanent relief and a healthier body, *we want to address the cause of the pain*. A good doctor or physical therapist can easily identify the cause of the pain. We often call this a diagnosis. The goal of forming a diagnosis is to address the cause of the problem.

When we see a person for his or her first visit in Physical Therapy, they are proud they have remembered the diagnosis the doctor gave them. "I have arthritis," they may say. Unfortunately, they may also fall into the trap of believing there is nothing that can be done for arthritis. This is not true. Often the diagnosis and the potential or ability to heal are not directly related. If 10 people are suffering from arthritis in their lower back, they may have 10 different responses in physical therapy.

When we handle the cause of the pain, we know it, because we experience long term, permanent relief and can get back to the activities we want to do.

"Back to Normal" Truth #3:

We have a choice in how we handle pain.

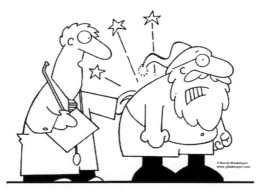

"The next time you lift someone's spirits, lift with your LEGS, not your BACK!"

Example: The Stained Ceiling Tile and the Leaky Roof

From Chapter 1, you realize we are constantly receiving information from different indicators.

In an office building I used to work in, we had a small leak in the ceiling in the middle of the gym. The leak did not seem to do much damage, but it always left an ugly, brown stain in the white ceiling tile. I noted that it only leaked when it rained hard and was windy at the same time. If the weather brought heavy rain, snow, sleet, freezing rain, or even hail without wind...no leak.

After changing the ceiling tile out 3 or 4 times, I climbed a ladder, pulled the ceiling tiles to the side and tried to find where the leak was coming from.

I am a Physical Therapist for a reason...and fixing leaks is not my God-given ability. No luck. I called a roofing company. They flooded the roof with 500 gallons...no leak. The roofing company reported that it was most likely coming from the heating and cooling units on the roof.

The HVAC company made some changes. No change...the small leak continued whenever the weather brought heavy rain and a strong wind. 3 roofing companies and 10 ceiling tiles later...the leak persisted. It was obvious what my choices were:

First, I could have ignored the problem all together and left the stained ceiling tile up. Ignoring the problem is usually not the best choice as it often leads to bigger problems down the road.

Second, I could have tried to alter or change the information. In fact, by changing the ceiling tile after every leak, that is exactly what I was doing. Was I addressing the cause of the leak? NO.

The third option was to address the cause. Then again, if you have ever tried to find a leak on a 4,000 square foot flat roof...the cause can be difficult to find.

There is a happy ending to the story as a roofer named Brian was performing other maintenance on the roof and found the cause of the leak. He patched it up and saved me lots of time climbing up ladders and a small fortune in ceiling tiles!

Applying Truth #3.

Working with a wide range of people in the PT clinic, we have noticed general truths in a person's health and how they handle problems with the body:

Healthy people address pain as soon as possible.
Unhealthy people ignore pain or try to alter it.

This is no different for any area in our life. Have you ever ignored a problem and it magically went away? That would be rare. Relationships, marriages, finances, health or the conditions of our life rarely get better when we ignore it.

In your case, if you have back pain and sciatica you can:

1. Ignore it. "Oh, it will go away in a day or two." There are many excuses we can come up with to explain away pain. Regardless, you have a problem and it should be addressed, especially if you plan on staying active in the future.

2. Try to change it. You can sit in a hot tub, use a heating pad, take an anti-inflammatory medicine or try to block the pain in a variety of other ways. Often you may do this together with "taking it easy" for a few days. Usually, the inflammation and pain decrease. Yet the pain will likely come back. Why? The cause has not been handled.

You may also change how you do certain movements. Usually we say a person is *compensating* when they do this.

If your pain increases when you sit...then logically, you may lean to the left to take pressure off of your right side.

3. Handle it. You wait a week. The pain is a little better, but continues to bother you with sitting. In the beginning, the pain was shooting down your leg to your ankle. Now it goes from your right buttocks to your knee. You call your physical therapist and make an appointment to get the problem handled.

As PTs, we are a little biased to #3. Then again, we have seen people suffer with lower back pain for more than 50 years prior to seeking treatment!

Questions for You:

1. What signs or information in your life have you ignored? What was the result?

2. Can you think of a time you ignored a problem and it went away on its own...and stayed away?

3. What examples can you think of when a person may change or alter their signs and information they are receiving?

4. Think of a person who is good at handling problems of the body. How is their overall health?

CHAPTER 5

What is the most common mistake people make in handling PAIN?

The easiest thing to do in any situation is to do nothing. It takes very little effort to make excuses as to why we have problems. It takes effort to face the problem and handle it.

A wise quote is, "We spend split seconds making decisions and spend the rest of our lives justifying them."

This happens with pain frequently. We feel back pain doing an everyday activity such as lifting something around the house or turning the wrong way. We are convinced we only have a "muscle spasm" and it will go away in a day or two...

A week later, the pain is still there. We have not done much all week, as moving the wrong way hurts.

Now we justify that we must have a bad back...just like our Uncle Barry. And we sit at work all day. And we never got around to getting back in shape like we were going to...

And we are carrying a few extra pounds in the front...

And we had an injury playing sports when we were younger. And...

While our egos are jumping at any reason to justify why we are in pain, <u>we are doing nothing at all to address the cause</u>.

By far the easiest thing to do in handling pain, is to ignore it...and make a load of excuses as to why we will not heal...and not get better.

It takes less effort to come up with excuses than to actually handle the cause of the problem. Not much less, but definitely less.

This brings us to "Back to Normal" Truth #4:

The most common mistake people make in handling pain is they IGNORE it.

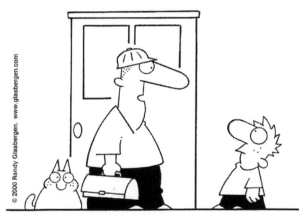

"What do we make where I work?
Mostly we make excuses."

If you want to make an excuse as to why you are unable to heal and will live the rest of your life in pain, feel free to choose from the list of my favorites:

10. "My _____ had the same problem." (fill in the blank with mom, dad, sister, brother, uncle or other relative...what do they have to do with you anyhow!?)

9. "I've always had a bad _____ " (fill in with back, neck, knee, shoulder, hip, ankle).

8. "I have arthritis."

7. "I have fibromyalgia."

6. "I don't have time...I'm too busy."

5. "My body is different than everyone else's...there is something wrong with me."

4. "It's an old injury...nothing can be done about it now."

3. "I have already tried everything."

2. "I do Physical Therapy already...I got exercises off the internet."

1. "I had an MRI and I have a bulging disc."

Look, you should expect to heal. We'll repeat that just to clarify...YOU SHOULD EXPECT TO HEAL.

How is that? If you were in the kitchen and accidentally cut your finger and had a small bleed, how long would you expect to keep bleeding? If you put a band-aid on the cut and took it off three days later, would you expect to see the cut still bleeding? Of course not! See, caught you expecting to heal...

The fact is 97% of your body is completely new from a year ago.

New nails, new hair, new skin.

You are constantly making a new you.

You are constantly healing. Regardless of your history, your family's history, or your present situation, you are healing. If you are breathing and your heart is beating, there is a really good chance you are healing.

Have you ever gone on a long walk and felt sore a day or two later? How long did that last? See, caught you healing again! If you do a new activity, one that you are not used to, you probably will be sore a day or two later from the muscle breakdown. Your body heals and you actually become stronger than before! Constant healing...

What Most People Do Throughout Life...

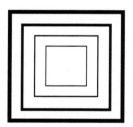 This diagram represents all of the activities a person may do in their day-to-day living. The outer boxes represent activities which require more strength, more energy, more flexibility, more health and more endurance such as running, twisting, and lifting. The inner boxes represent lighter, easier activities such as sitting or lying down.

This is typically what happens when we ignore the problem of pain: In our 20's and 30's, we likely experience very little long lasting, debilitating pain. We can help a friend move, do hours of yardwork and walk a few miles with minimal problems. Maybe we have a little soreness the day after, but it does not last long. Our ability to heal is high at this point in our life. It is only when we lift something very heavy or run or perform some other high intensity activity that we have pain. At this age, with the inflammation resolving in a day or two, we convince ourselves to ignore the pain. "It will go away." We will just be a little more careful next time.

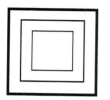 Eventually, as we move into our 40's, we stop lifting heavy objects or running altogether. Now, we begin having pain if we do too many stairs or walk a few miles. We now need to take a break as we are driving the 4 hour trip to the shore for vacation. As long as we continue to ignore our problem, it continues to get worse. We eventually begin compensating when we walk or take the stairs. "This is just part of my age," we may reason.

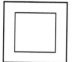 In our 50's, we may start leaning on the grocery cart to help us make it through the trip to the local grocery store. Standing for anything longer than 30 minutes is now tough. We begin taking breaks any time we sit, stand, or walk for a few minutes. It now takes an hour or so for the stiffness to go away when we get up in the morning. Getting dressed in the morning is a real challenge. "I'm getting old."

 In our 60's and 70's, we may now be facing total joint replacements and looking for any sort of relief as the pain is with us for most activities. The only time we are not in pain is when we are sitting in our favorite recliner or lying down. We are now boxed in living our life through only a few basic activities.

Where did we go wrong? Why is it that some people stay very active into their 90's and beyond and others can barely move in their 50's?

Is it genetics? Maybe that plays a small part.

Is it a magic pill? Doubtful, as large populations of people around the world stay active and have minimal arthritis without the latest multivitamin or wonder drug.

It is most likely the way we prevent and handle problems as they happen in the body.

Ignore it and you likely will lose most of the activities you want to do. Handle it and you can still be dancing well into your 90's and beyond.

Questions for You:

1. Think of the worst pain you have felt in the past year.
2. How did you handle the pain?
3. Did you ignore it, change it or handle it?

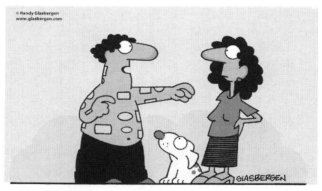

"One patch makes me stop smoking, one makes me eat less, one makes me put my clothes in the hamper instead of leaving them on the floor, one makes me put the toilet seat back down..."

What is the Best Treatment for YOUR Pain?

You can walk into any pharmacy or supermarket and find a gazillion different treatments for pain. The latest gadgets and gizmos for back pain are available on TV...if you want to stay up until 3 in the morning. Famous basketball and football players endorse blue creams and heat packs for joint pain. The number of treatment options can be overwhelming *if you do not know how to sort through the mess*.

Here is a list of a few treatments for back and joint pain:

- Heat
- Ice
- Medicine (anti-inflammatories, muscle relaxants, pain killers)
- Surgery
- Injections
- Herbal remedies
- Joint juice
- Vitamins and supplements (glucosamine)
- Massage
- Physical Therapy
- Exercise
- Chiropractic
- Electric Stimulation
- Ultrasound
- Laser
- Sports Creams

From the Truths we have covered so far, you know that the only way for you to get back to normal is to handle the CAUSE of your back pain and sciatica...

Fortunately, for the guy who throws his back out and would rather just find the best possible treatment now instead of testing every product in Aisle 9 at CVS, there is a quick, easy answer: RESEARCH.

Specifically...RESEARCH on what has worked for other people who have the same CAUSE of back pain and sciatica as you do.

In Physical Therapy, we use research to select the best treatments for you. What has worked for thousands of others with similar pain and the same CAUSE as your problem, will likely work for you.

For example, in the treatment of back and neck pain, 3 things have stood the test of time. We will discuss what works in the next chapter...

Questions for You:

1. What treatments have you tried in the past?
2. Were they pretending to help? Or were they truly helping?
3. Do you still have the pain now?

What is the Best Treatment for YOU?

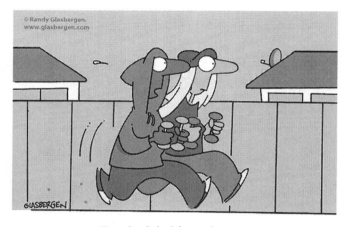

"Running is bad for my knees.
Not running is bad for everything else!"

3 Treatments have stood the test of time for lower back pain and neck pain:

1. **Exercise.**
2. **Manual therapy.** (also known as Hands-on, mobilization or manipulation).
3. **Traction.**

Exercise.

Remember back in the 1950's and 60's? What was the standard treatment for lower back pain? BED REST. Days upon days, which turned into weeks upon weeks of bed rest.

Back strain?
BED REST.
Back spasm?
BED REST.
Herniated disc?
BED REST.
Arthritis?
BED REST.

Sounds exciting...huh?

Well, luckily we now know that bed rest is actually likely to cause more harm than good. The latest research shows that one of the best things we can do for back pain is to keep moving!

Why does exercise work?

When our back is painful and inflamed, we have damaged tissue. Damaged tissue is painful. If we do not move, healing is slow.

When we do move, even if it is light exercise or walking slowly, blood flow increases. This speeds up the healing process as damaged tissue is removed and the building blocks for new tissue is delivered to the injured area.

Think about this: Would you rather drink from a flowing, mountain stream or a mud puddle? And not just any mud puddle, but the kind with mosquito eggs and bugs floating across the top?

Mountain streams are used in beverage commercials. Mud puddles are not.

Flowing is healthy. Still, cesspools are not healthy.

People moving are healthy. People sleeping on recliners and not moving are not.

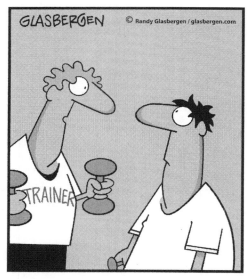

"If you haven't exercised in a while,
you may need to stretch and warm up
before you stretch and warm up."

What is the best exercise for your back or neck pain?

Not all exercises treat the same problem. As we will cover in the next chapter, there are three common causes of back pain and three common causes of neck pain.

The key is to do the right exercises that are the right ones for your problem.

Here's the deal with exercise...
There are 2 types of exercise that work:

1. Corrective exercise. Several exercise systems exist for the sole purpose of providing relief and correcting bad habits.

2. Strengthening. Most people we see for back pain and sciatica do stretching exercises...and that's fine. It can give temporary relief.

However, long term, we want to focus on strengthening...and what this does is retrain the muscle and improve stability so your pain doesn't come back in the future...

Hands-on Physical Therapy.

Manual therapy goes by several different names: mobilization, manipulation, and hands-on therapy are the most common.

Regardless of the exact word, the concept is that the therapist is using a hands-on technique to help you move better.

The concept is this: A person comes in with pain every time they bend backwards. They feel "blocked". The therapist may do a hands-on technique to help them move through the barrier. This is usually pain free and results in an immediate improvement.

Traditionally, chiropractors are known for this.

Hands-on therapy works. When we restore normal movement in the joint and then do exercises to retrain the muscle which controls the joint, something neat can happen...long term, permanent relief.

A Word of Caution

Some people get on the Manual Therapy Roller Coaster. Every time their back goes out or they have a "crick" in the neck, they run and get manual therapy. The key to preventing that from coming back is exercise.

Also, people who only exercise without receiving manual therapy, at least initially, often end up only retraining bad movement patterns and may experience only limited relief with exercise.

Formula for Permanent Relief:

Manual Therapy to Restore Normal Movement
+
Exercise to Retrain the Muscles

Traction

Traction, or its close relative Decompression, is effective for a few types of back or neck pain.

The first is arthritis (which is similar to disc degeneration and stenosis). With arthritis, the bones (called "vertebrae") in the spine become closer together. Traction is effective at improving this space and preventing the problem from getting worse.

The second type of problem traction works well with is sciatica. This is when pain shoots down into the leg. This is tricky, as the cause of the problem is not in the leg...but in the back.

"Back to Normal" Truth #5:

The most effective treatments for lower back pain and sciatica are hands-on treatment, exercise and traction.

Successful treatment involves your physical therapist finding the cause of your problem and then using the right combination of exercise, manual therapy and traction to handle that problem and help you heal.

At the end of this book, we have given you some basic exercises to get you started...but for the best chances of successful treatment, schedule an appointment and come see one of our Back Pain & Sciatica Specialists at Madden Physical Therapy.

Please send Chad an email at **chad.madden@maddenpt.com** – we would love to get you scheduled and well on your way Back to Normal!

Success Stories

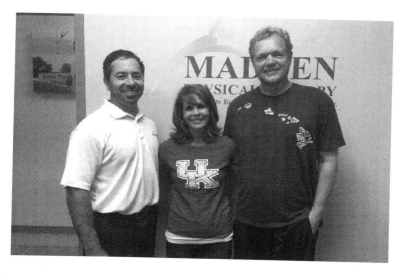

Chad Madden, PT; Grace & Ken Vanwingerden, Happy Madden Graduates

Flying in from Kentucky for Back Treatment

❝ *I've had back pain for years. I've seen 3 orthopedic surgeons... 2 recommend surgery. I was on pain killers...for the first time in my life. And I started doing research on the internet. I wanted to know if there was something else out there other than pain pills and surgery...trying to figure out what to do to get relief.*

I found Chad's videos online...and he made it sound like this was really simple to take care of. We spoke on the phone...and I took the leap of faith to fly in from Lexington, Kentucky to Harrisburg for treatment. It was a little bit of a challenge. Sure enough, I'm walking out of here in disbelief... It's a shocking difference... He completely fixed it...I have complete relief. I've been to other PTs...and I'm not sure why everyone else isn't treating like this... All I know is this works...and I'm flying back again...if I need it."

— Ken Vanwingerden

Lexington, KY

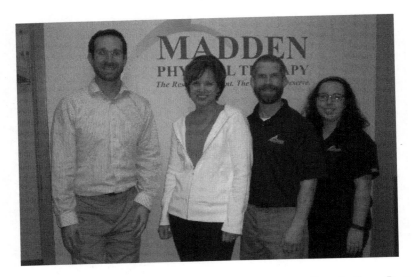

Andrew Dulak, DPT; happy Madden PT patient, Susan Barrett; Ryan Barr, PTA; Heather Purcell, PT Aide

❝ *Prior to coming here, I had severe pain in the morning upon getting out of bed. My sciatic nerve pain prevented me from sitting, standing, walking for long periods of time & I had to stop golfing. I had back surgery in July 2014, but did not have PT afterwards. I returned to golfing summer of 2015, but had to stop in July due to pain. My PT plan has been fantastic. I truly feel 99% better & the best I have felt since surgery."*

— Susan Barrett

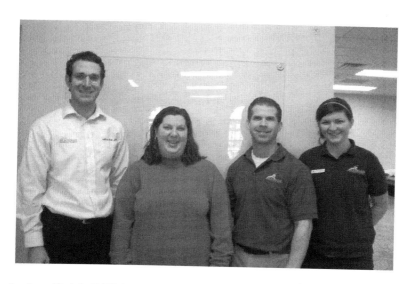

Andrew Dulak, DPT; happy Madden PT patient, Angel Scully; Ryan Barr, PTA; Justina Malehorn, PT Aide

❝ *I am very happy with my results from physical therapy. Before I came, I didn't have major pain all the time, but I kept doing everyday activities that would cause a flare-up. That doesn't happen anymore. I had a lot of trouble getting dressed, rolling over in bed hurt, and sitting at work all day was uncomfortable. I am 100% better than when I started here. The staff was all great to deal with from the office staff to Justina, Ryan, & Andrew. My experience was great, thank you all for helping me get better."*

— **Angel Scully**

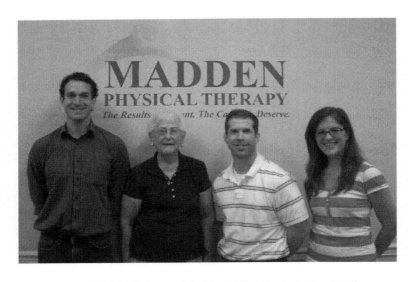

*Andrew Dulak, DPT; happy Madden PT patient, Catherine Sener;
Ryan Barr, PTA; Janel Wolfe, PT Aide*

❝ *What would I have done without them! They were all great.
I hurt so badly when I came here. After my falls I could do very little.
I cancelled several appointments my pain was so bad I couldn't get on
the table. Now I'm back to walking daily and ready to go back to 'Silver
Sneakers' program. I have a slight problem with my right ankle, which I'm
sure will get better. They all were so great and patient with me, but
I hope I never have to see them as a patient."*

— **Catherine Sener**

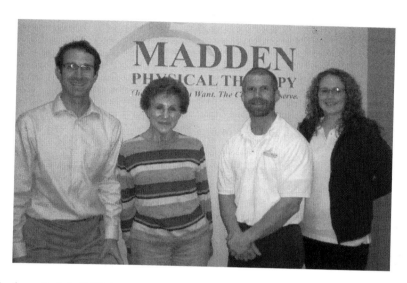

Andrew Dulak, DPT; happy Madden PT patient, Rachel Springer; Ryan Barr, PTA; Victoria Motz, PT Aide

❝ *I love the one-on-one experience. You are told if you are doing your exercises wrong. I had severe back pain even walking 5 minutes. Now I can walk without any pain. I admit, I was doubtful because I had tried other PT elsewhere & it was not working. I am thrilled that I can avoid more surgery at this point. I will faithfully do the exercises at home. The cards are a great help. All in all, it has been a wonderful experience."*

— **Rachel Springer**

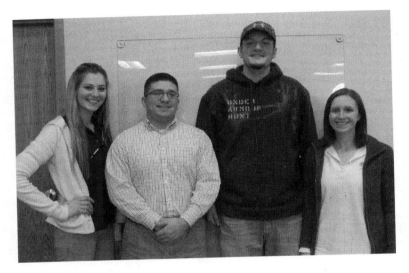

*Tiffany Todd, PT Aide; Dan Hinnerschitz, DPT; happy Madden PT patient,
Bob D.; Amanda Milliron, PTA*

❝ *When I first started having issues with my lower back and
shooting pains down my leg, I was very skeptical about coming to PT.
I was at another PT office 2 years ago when the first incident occurred
and it was a waste of my time. They didn't listen to what I was trying to
tell them about my pain. When I came here to Madden, Dan, Amanda,
and Tiffany paid attention when I would tell them about my pain. They
made a workout that took my pain away within two weeks. I couldn't be
happier with my experience and will be sure to refer anyone I know who
needs PT to come to Madden."*

— **Bob D.**

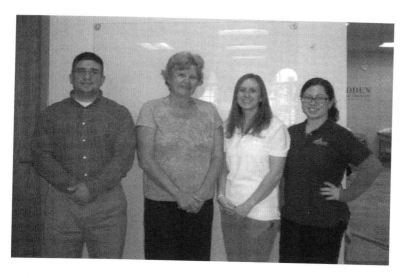

Dan Hinnerschitz, DPT; happy Madden PT patient, Dee R.; Amanda Milliron, PTA; Kate Dunn, PT Aide

❝ *I am very pleased with the resolution of my back and sciatic pain. I had unrelenting pain down my leg before starting PT. The exercises and stretching by Dan gave slow but steady relief from the pain. I can now do my daily activities, including babysitting my 10 month old granddaughter, without pain. Thanks Dan, Amanda, Kate, and Emily!"*

— Dee R.

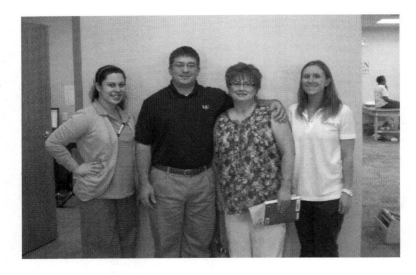

Kate Dunn, PT Aide; Dan Hinnerschitz, DPT; happy Madden PT patient, Suzi H.; Amanda Milliron, PTA

❝ *I came for therapy because I had quite an increase in pain both in my back and with chronic sciatica. I rarely could sleep through the night because of the severe pain. Most of my daily activities had to be sharply curtailed. I've seen a real improvement not only in my ability to resume my daily routine, but also being able to get a good night's sleep!*

The staff here is wonderful–They're knowledgeable and personable at the same time. There was never a day that I came when they weren't in a good mood, upbeat, and ready to help me do the best I could. I would definitely come back if necessary."

— **Suzi H.**

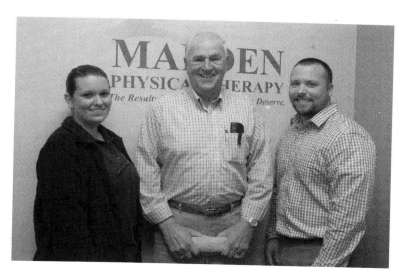

Bethany Holt, PT Aide; happy Madden PT patient, Glen M.; Joe Hribick, DPT

❝ *When I came here I had extreme pain in my lower back and down my right leg. After my time at Madden, I am basically pain-free. I still need to do my daily exercises to keep from going backwards to my previous problems. The staff here at Madden has been very helpful and understanding. Jim Glass referred me to Madden and I wanted to say thanks to him as well for the wonderful referral. Joe (my therapist) was very patient with me throughout my whole treatment and I thank you!"*

— Glen "Bud" M.

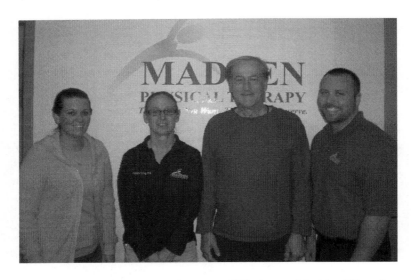

Bethany Holt, PT Aide; Michelle Young, PTA; happy Madden PT patient, Jonathan W.; Joe Hribick, DPT

❝ *It has been a long time since I have experienced in the health industry the care, professionalism, and empathy by all the staff here at Madden. From the receptionists, to the Patient Liaison, to especially all of the Physical Therapists. They have always been supportive and friendly. Since this is my last day, I hate to leave, but all the PT has helped me get better and relieve the pain. Thank you all, especially Michelle, Dan, and of course Joe."*

— **Jonathan W.**

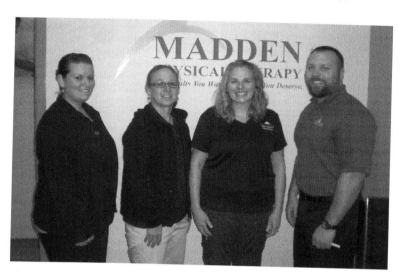

Bethany Holt, PT Aide; Michelle Young, PTA; happy Madden PT patient, Jamie S.; Joe Hribick, DPT

❝ Before coming to PT at Madden, there were days I barely could get through the day without wanting to cry from pain. As an OT in pediatrics, my job is for me to be mobile and it was getting increasingly difficult. There were also days where heavy lifting/work caused me difficulty even getting out of bed. Since coming to PT and working with Joe and Michelle, there are days, more so than not, where I think, "I can't believe another day of no pain." They have given me the ability to do my job better, be an active participant in my life, and know what a pain-free life means. The tools they have provided me have made me successful and excited as I continue my life and my passion of working with kids with no pain. I am forever grateful for the wonderful experience. Thank you!"

— **Jamie S.**

Top 3 Home Exercises
for Pelvic Pain

1. Single Knee Isometric

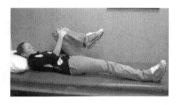

How to do it:
1. Lying on your back, grab your knee with both hands.
2. Keep your other leg straight.
3. Push your knee down into your hands.
4. Keep breathing.

Hold 5 seconds, 10 times.
DO NOT hug your knee to your chest!

What does it do?
This exercise fires muscles in your buttocks and helps half of the pelvis rock in one direction.

2. Ball Squeeze

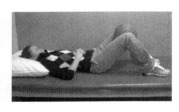

How to do it:
1. Lying on your back with knees bent.
2. Ball between the knees.
3. Slightly arch your back by pressing your buttocks into the table. Slightly tighten your stomach muscles.

4. Squeeze the ball.
5. Keep breathing. DO NOT bear down or strain.

Hold 10 seconds, repeat 10 times.

No Ball?
A pillow off of your couch or a folded pillow will work just fine!

3. Knees Apart with Band

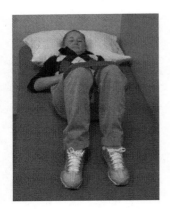

How to do it:
1. Lying on your back with knees bent.
2. Band around knees.
3. Slightly arch your back by pressing your buttocks into the table. Slightly tighten your stomach muscles.
4. Spread knees apart.
5. Keep breathing. DO NOT bear down or strain.

Hold 5 seconds, repeat 20 times.

Top 3 Home Exercises
for Herniated Discs in the Lower Back and SCIATICA

1. Prop-Up on Stomach

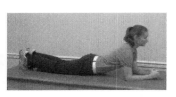

How to do it:
1. Lying on your stomach, prop up on your elbows.
2. Keep breathing.

Hold for up to 2 minutes.

Too Hard? Try This ...
1. Same position.
2. Lay on a pillow under your chest with arms at your side.

What Should I feel?
If your pain is coming from a herniated disc, you should feel less pain in your legs and more in your lower back.

2. Press-Up on Stomach

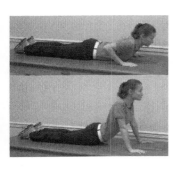

How to do it:
1. Lying on your stomach, hands in push-up position.
2. Keep hips and pelvis on floor, press upper body, head and chest up.

Hold 5 seconds, repeat 10 times.

Too Hard? Try This ...

Instead of placing hands underneath shoulders, move them forward or up 6 inches and decrease how much you bend back.

3. Standing Back Bend

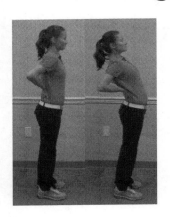

How to do it:

1. Standing with hands placed on the small of your back.

2. Bend backwards.

Repeat 20 times.

Top 3 Home Exercises
for Arthritis in the Lower Back

1. Trunk Rotation

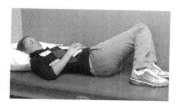

How to do it:
1. Lying on your back with knees bent. Feet on the mat or bed.
2. Keep shoulder blades on the mat and feet and knees together.
3. Rotate knees to the right side.
4. Then to the left.

Alternate right, then left. 20 times each side.

Good Idea!
For those with early morning back stiffness, this works well before getting out of bed.

2. Double Knees to Chest

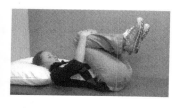

How to do it:
1. Lying on your back, hug both knees toward your chest.
2. Keep breathing.

Hold 5 seconds, repeat 10 times.

If hugging your knees is too difficult, wrap a towel or belt behind the knees and pull to chest.

Why It Works:
This movement increases the space between the bones in your back.

3. Single Knee to Chest

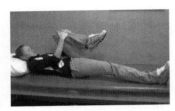

How to do it:
1. Lying on your back, hug one knee toward your chest.
2. Keep other leg straight down.
3. Keep breathing.

Hold 5 seconds, repeat 10 times on each leg.

A Special Offer for You... the Reader of "Back to Normal"

So after reading this book..."Back to Normal"...we're offering you help...but only if you want it.

Are you looking for permanent relief without medications, injections and surgery?

Sometimes this is super easy...

Other times it can be more complicated.

If you're looking for more tools to heal naturally without medications, injections or surgery...send me an email at **chad.madden@maddenpt.com**.

In the subject line write what you think the cause of your pain is. ("Stenosis"; or "Herniated Disc"; or "SI Joint")

Then in the email...let me know why you think that's your cause.

I check my email a few times a day...and will get back to you with some helpful advice as soon as possible.

Cordially,

Chad Madden
Physical Therapist, Back Pain & Sciatica Specialist

The Real Story About the Founder of Madden Physical Therapy...

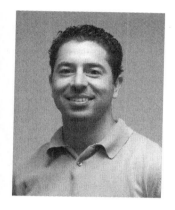

Hi. This is Chad Madden.

For years, I've offered up a vanilla, professional, super-safe Bio...and I have it for you below...(just in case that's what you're looking for...)

If you're looking for more though...the real dirt on me...I've gone out on a limb and revealed that for you as well...

Chad Madden is the Founder of Madden Physical Therapy and #1 Most Watched Back Pain and Sciatica Specialist in the World.

He grew up in West Hanover and graduated from Central Dauphin High School in 1995. He enjoyed a mediocre sports career in football, wrestling and track.

Realizing his strengths were in academics...and not sports...he earned his Master's Degree in Physical Therapy at College Misericordia in Dallas, PA (outside of Wilkes-Barre). There he played 4 years of baseball...cementing his legacy as a mediocre athlete.

On September 2, 2003, he opened Madden Physical Therapy with a total staff of one Receptionist...in a 2,000 square foot clinic on Prince Street. His oldest son was born 3 days later on September 5th...(Good timing!)

Chad's treatment schedule is limited today as he focuses much of his time and energy working with and helping other Physical Therapy owners across the US and Australia. He is the co-Founder of that company... Breakthrough PT Marketing.

Chad presently lives in East Hanover on a 3 acre farmette with his wife, Stephanie, their 5 children (4 boys and a girl), 5 mini donkeys, 7 chickens, 2 cats and a one-eyed Border Collie, Georgia. In their spare time...just kidding...there is no spare time.

So that's it...see...I warned you...pretty vanilla.

Now the REAL Juicy Stuff...

First, I'm a Bethlehem Steel Baby...

That means my parents met at Bethlehem Steel...and likely conceived me there.

They were young...and made it work.

How young? (My grandmother was 35 when I was born).

They have another son too...my brother...Steve.

Rather than share all the dirt on Steve...I'll just say that for years I introduced myself as "Steve Madden's brother."

In comparison, I was fairly introverted growing up...read a lot of books... especially Encyclopedia Brown and the Hardy Boys.

(I still read a ton today....and have 500+ books in my office...my favorites are a handful of Classics from the late, great Charlie "Tremendous" Jones...)

On to sports...I love them...

I just never made a team I tried out for...

5 feet 8 inches...not fast...and skinny is a bad combination...

And frankly, I was just not that good...

In spite of my athletic shortcomings, I played 17 years of baseball, 6 years of basketball, 9 years of football, 3 years of track, wrestled for 2 years... and oh, yeah, played the saxophone and drums.

Why am I telling you this?

Well one of those years, playing football for the Linglestown Colts, Rodney Krasevic tackled me...and I broke my left collar bone.

Back in the day, there wasn't rehab for a 13 year old with a collar bone fracture...just a butterfly brace for 4 weeks...then go back and play.

Well that didn't work well...even a few months later...I still didn't feel 100%...nor even close to it.

So after missing the basketball team at East Jr., it gave me a chance to start lifting weights...

And I noticed immediate changes to my 120 pound body...good changes.

And I saw that lifting and training could change a body.

The seed was planted.

So at this time, I'm pretty much a nerdy bookworm type who was good at science and math who just discovered weight training...

And by the time high school rolled around...I started focusing in on engineering...and taking engineering classes at Central Dauphin HS.

I need to give MAJOR credit to my guidance counselor at CD...Dale Houck...who helped me through some soul searching my Sophomore year...

At the time, the engineer work and career didn't really appeal to me...I wanted to work more with people.

He recognized this (you know how lousy most 16 year old semi-rebellious boys are at clearly communicating...)

And recommended I start volunteering in a Physical Therapy clinic...to see if that resonated with what I felt my purpose was.

So I did.

And I started volunteering with Dale Hilbolt at 899 S. Arlington Avenue.

Dale was an awesome mentor and helped tremendously to really shape my early PT career.

After volunteering with Dale...I knew Physical Therapy was what I wanted to do.

Routinely, I'll hear from people who come through Madden PT for treatment, "Wow...I remember when you were back on Prince Street... you've really come a long way."

And I'll share the same thing with you that I've shared with them:

"The success is a reflection of 3 types of people in my life: People like Dale who helped me in the beginning...World Class staff who care...and the clients we have the privilege and honor to serve everyday."

Speaking of the important people who nurtured me early on...

We've seen a ton of clients who either knew or were initially referred in by my late grandparents...Polly and Jack Madden who lived on Virginia Avenue by the old Central Dauphin High School.

I can remember stopping in after school...grabbing a bowl of Cheez-Itz and a soda...and asking Grandma to wake me up in 11 minutes...so I could make it back in time for a game.

The other thing I clearly remember is Jack (my grandfather) sharing with me his stories of being a beer salesman and promoter for Wilsbach Distributors...and how, in his 37 years of service, **he never lost a customer.**

That was super important to him...

And it's something that really stuck with me.

After graduating from Central Dauphin in 1995, I received an academic scholarship to College Misericordia in Dallas, PA (the College is now called Misericordia University).

It was an ideal setting for me...small, kind of close to home...but far enough away where I could go through the "figure out who I am" phase.

I earned a Master's Degree in Physical Therapy in 2000...and a Bachelor's of Science Degree. In my time there I played baseball for 4 years and also was elected Captain my Senior year...and was the Assistant Coach my graduate year. And saying I was mediocre would be an overstatement.

After graduation and passing my Physical Therapy license exam...I first worked for Arlington Orthopedics. If memory serves me correct, the PT arm was called Arlington Rehabilitation and Sports Performance.

While I'm not a big fan of Physician Owned Physical Therapy practices... it was an ideal first job for me...and I did that for 2 years.

After that, I took a job as a Clinical Director with Dale's company...formerly known as First Choice.

In the end, it wasn't the right fit for me...and I really wanted to do my own thing.

So with my wife being 9 months pregnant (literally)...we opened Madden Physical Therapy on September 2, 2003.

My first son was born 3 days later...on September 5, 2003.

Not the best timing on my part...

But we made it work.

I'm not sure why my timing stunk so bad...I kept thinking if I didn't do something "Before my first child was born", I'd never do it.

I can distinctly remember cleaning the office and getting everything set up the day before we were to open (appropriately Labor Day)...and seeing Stephanie, my wife, have to take a break.

And thinking to myself, "Oh $#%&...I better make this work."

And being committed to doing so.

And it has worked...

The main reason being because we have great people...

Just this morning, the father of a patient stopped me in the parking lot and said, "Hey, I've been to a lot of other places...and you have the nicest place. Great people."

We put a lot of effort into creating a unique healing experience.

It hasn't always been easy or perfect....
But it's been an amazing journey.

If you've made it this far...I promised you I'd reveal some dirt...here it is:

1. My office is a mess.

I've been saying for 6 years now that I'm "reorganizing." Let's face it... my strength is in creating, not organizing. Right now, I have the #1 Videos in the world on YouTube for 6 different categories...created the Top 3 Program...am writing 3 books...led the creation of our one-of-a-kind Exercise Card System...so I'm creative. I'm not organized. But I'm surrounded with organized people.

2. I take on crazy BIG projects.

Someone recently said to me, "The thing I like about you is you pretend to act like you don't know what the limit is."

While that's true, it drives some people crazy. I'm an idea man...not necessarily grounded in what most people accept as status quo.

This makes some uncomfortable...yet Madden PT wouldn't be serving as many people as we are today...we wouldn't be having people fly in from Colorado or Montana or Kentucky for Physical Therapy...or wouldn't be coaching over 145 other Physical Therapy companies...if we would have accepted the self-limiting beliefs of others.

3. I'm almost always 3 minutes late...

Real World Update:

In spite of my flaws...my wife, Stephanie, and I now have 5 kids (4 sons and a daughter), 5 mini donkeys (Peppermint Patty, MoonBeam, Haley, Cactus Kate and Pistol Pete), 2 cats - Lucky & Charms, and a Border Collie named Georgia.

Because Stephanie runs a tight ship at the house...and because of our World Class staff...I've been given the opportunity to go out and help 100's of other Physical Therapists across the US and now in Australia (called "physios" in Australia).

I write 6 mornings per week...and study every night.

Our kids are super active...and both of our parents are supportive in helping us taxi and support.

And I'll leave you with this:

My favorite verse is, "The stone the builder's rejected has become the cap stone. The Lord has done this and it is beautiful in our eyes."

And I think that's a sound statement to represent my story...and probably your story as well.

So as I shared above, my World Class Team and I are super focused and committed to creating an Amazing Experience for the Clients we work with.

Are you looking for an Amazing Experience?

If you are...and you'd like to share your story...email me at **chad.madden@maddenpt.com**. In the subject line write "My Story".

When you do, I'll have a special gift just for you.

Looking forward to hearing from you,

Chad

PS - Again the easiest way to reach me is my email, **chad.madden@maddenpt.com**. *I'd love to hear your story...*

The Real Story of Daniel Hinnerschitz, Doctor of Physical Therapy

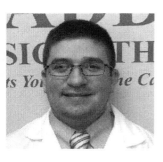

People always ask me how I became interested in physical therapy, well here you go...

Most folks had a prior experience with physical therapy, thought it was a pretty cool profession and went on to PT school. Well, not me...

I really didn't know anything about PT when I was a senior in high school and had to decide what I wanted to do for the rest of my life...

I was very interested in sports at the time and had been recruited to play football at Lebanon Valley College.

That's when coach Pantalone told me about the schools brand new physical therapy program.

I knew I wanted to do something with sports or health and wellness, and PT sounded like something I would be interested in... so I applied to the program, got accepted, and never looked back!

Long story short, I never ended up playing football in college...

Fast forward to 6 years later and I graduated from LVC with a Doctorate in Physical Therapy degree in 2012.

I sure am glad that I choose a career in physical therapy. It's great being in a position to help people heal naturally without requiring medications, injections, and surgery.

My favorite part about being a physical therapist is helping my patients get back to a normal life and getting them back to the activities they love doing the most.

It's a very rewarding career, and at the end of each day, I can say that I'm making a difference by being able to help people every day.

Here at Madden Physical Therapy, I specialize in using hands-on manual therapy to treat orthopedic conditions, especially of the spine.

My favorite thing to treat is lower back pain and sciatica.

On a personal level:

Here are some things I enjoy doing in my free time...

I enjoy travelling – I'm always on the go – whether I'm vacationing or just visiting family or some of my college buddies.

I was also fortunate enough to spend a semester in New Zealand when I was in undergraduate school in 2008.

I'm a HUGE sports fan...

Football is my favorite sport, but I enjoy watching most sporting events.

My favorite teams are Penn State, the Green Bay Packers, and the New York Mets.

Finally, I enjoy spending time outdoors and especially enjoy going for hikes.

The Real Story of Joe Hribick, Doctor of Physical Therapy

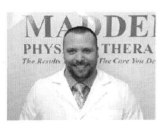

So I grew up in Lititz, PA and got my Doctorate of Physical Therapy degree from Lebanon Valley College in 2011.

I also work as an adjunct instructor at LVC teaching physical therapy doctorate students how to perform hands-on techniques.

My education and PT schooling was certainly my #1 priority...

I was Valedictorian of my class, was nominated for the American Physical Therapy Association's Outstanding Physical Therapy Student Award, and was the recipient of the Academic Achievement Award for my class.

Taking it back even further... ever since I was young, I knew I wanted to choose a career where I could make a difference in the lives of others each day.

I was strong in science and math, and grew up playing several sports.

I have always been passionate about physical fitness and helping others live a healthy life...

So naturally, the profession of Physical Therapy fit me like a glove!

I love hearing my patients tell me how physical therapy has helped them get their lives back... and I especially love being able to make an immediate change in someone's pain on their first visit and show them that their condition CAN truly be helped.

Outside of work:

I love spending time with my wife, Emily, and family... we are always running from one event to the next around the holidays to fit in time with everyone!

We recently bought our first home in Mount Joy, PA.

And actually, Emily is a Physical Therapist, too – but she specializes in Pediatrics (working with children)... and she is quite good at it.

I enjoy being very physically active and spend a lot of time outdoors doing fun, thrill-seeking stuff like mountain biking, trail running, backpacking, skiing, and competing in off-road triathlons.

What I like most though...is being able to share my experiences with family and friends.

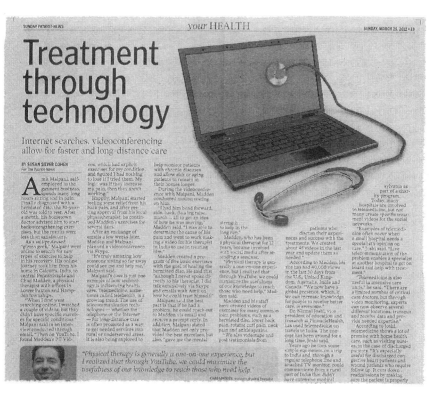

As seen in The Patriot-News
on Sunday, March 25, 2012.

❝ Amit Malpani, self-employed in the garment business, spends many long hours sitting and in pain. Finally diagnosed with a herniated disc, the 30-year-old was told to rest. After a month, his hometown doctor advised him to start back-strengthening exercises, but the results were less than satisfactory.

As a self-professed "gizmo geek," Malpani went online to search for new types of exercise to help in his recovery. His online journey took him from his home in Calcutta, India, to

73

central Pennsylvania and Chad Madden, a physical therapist with offices in Lower Paxton and Hampden townships.

"When I first went searching online, I watched a couple of videos, but they didn't have specific exercises for specific conditions," Malpani said in an interview conducted through email. "Then on YouTube, I found Madden's PT Videos, which had explicit exercises for my condition, and figured I had nothing to lose if I tried them. My logic was if they increase my pain, then they aren't working."

Happily, Malpani started feeling some relief from his back pain, and after getting approval from his local physiotherapist, he continued Madden's exercises for several days.

After an exchange of emails a few weeks later, Madden and Malpani planned a videoconference via Skype.

"It's truly amazing how someone sitting so far away could see me and help me," Malpani said.

Malpani's case is just one example of how technology is influencing health care. Telemedicine, sometimes called telehealth, is a growing trend. The use of telecommunication technologies – whether the telephone or the internet – for long-distance care is often promoted as a way to get needed services into rural or underserved areas. It is also being explored to help monitor patients with chronic diseases and allow sick or aging patients to remain in their homes longer.

During the videoconference with Malpani, Madden conducted motion testing on him.

"I had him bend forward, side, back, do a leg raise, march... all to get an idea of how he was moving," Madden said. "I was able to determine the cause of his pain and went to work making a video for his therapist in India to use in treating him."

Madden created a program of five basic exercises with the goal of healing the herniated disc. He said that "although I never spoke directly to his therapist, I did talk extensively via Skype and emails with Amit on how he could treat himself."

Malpani said the best part is that if he had a problem, he could reach out to Madden via email and receive a prompt reply. In addition, Malpani stated that Madden not only provided the best exercises, but also, "gave me the mental strength to help in the long run."

Madden, who has been a physical therapist for 12 years, became involved with social media after attending a seminar.

"Physical therapy is generally a one-on-one experience, but I realize that through YouTube, we could maximize the usefulness of our knowledge to reach those who need help," Madden said.

Madden and his staff have created videos of exercises for many common joint problems, such as a herniated disc, lower back pain, rotator cuff pain, neck pain and ankle sprains.

"We also videotape and post testimonials from patients who discuss their experiences and success with the treatments. We created about 45 videos in the last year and update them as needed."

According to Madden, his site has had 40,000 views in the last 30 days from the U.S., United Kingdom, Australia, India and Canada. "We now have a global presence, which, if we can increase knowledge for people to receive better care, is awesome."

Dr. Nirmal Joshi, vice president of education and research at PinnacleHealth, has used telemedicine on travels to India. The concept has been around for a long time, Joshi said.

Years ago he took some simple equipment on a trip to India and, through a regular telephone line and attached TV monitor, could communicate from a rural part of India that didn't have extensive medical care, to specialists in Pennsylvania as part of a charity program. Today, many hospitals are involved in telemedicine, but not many create specific treatment videos for the social networks.

"Examples of telemedicine often occur when a small hospital needs a specialist's opinion on care," Joshi said. "Live telecommunication of the problem enables a specialist at another hospital to get on board and help with treatment."

"Telemedicine is also useful in intensive care units," he said.

"There are a limited number of critical care doctors, but through video monitoring, experts can now observe several different locations, transmit and receive data and provide needed expertise."

According to Joshi, telemedicine shows a lot of promise with home health care, such as visiting nurses, in the case of discharged congestive heart patients and wound patients who require follow up. It cuts down readmissions by making sure the patient is properly healing."

99

Made in the USA
Columbia, SC
20 August 2018